Living With A Diabetic Dog

How To Keep Your Dog Healthy, Prevent Common Problems And Avoid Complications

by

Amy Newton Thomas and Bruce Pea

Table of Contents

Preface

This book is for informational purposes only. I am not a veterinary doctor and I am not providing veterinary medical advice of any kind for anyone or any dog.

Please consult your veterinarian before doing anything that may affect your dogs health.

What I am offering are useful lessons I've learned living day-to-day with Willie, my diabetic dog. I want to share insights I've learned that have helped me manage Willie's diabetes better and improve both our day-to-day lives.

If your dog was recently diagnosed with diabetes, this book will provide helpful information for both you and your dog.

If you are already living with a diabetic dog, you will discover useful tips to improve both you and your dog's lifestyle.

And please, always talk with your veterinarian before doing anything that could affect your dogs health and well being.

"Your Dog Has Diabetes"

The veterinarian's tone was matter-of-fact and his words were spoken without emotion, "I'm rushing your dog to the university vet-med hospital for emergency surgery!" I was attending a conference and had boarded Willie, my twelve year old Pembroke Welsh Corgi, with his vet. The cryptic message on my cell phone left my head spinning and my stomach turning.

What happened? Willie was fine when I dropped him off two days earlier.

I replayed the message a couple more times then called the veterinarian. He said Willie had twisted his stomach and needed emergency surgery right away to fix the problem.

How does that happen? Did he fall? Get into a fight with another dog?

I told the veterinarian I was on my way home and would go directly to the university vet-med hospital as soon as I got to town.

I arrived at the vet-med hospital and was immediately taken to the veterinarian treating Willie who took me to the emergency room. Willie was lying on a stainless steel table that felt as cold and hard as it looked. The high intensity

2

light made him look flat and two-dimensional. He was sprawled out like a rag doll, surrounded by vet techs, completely unresponsive.

He looked awful.

The veterinarian pulled me aside and said they had examined Willie and ran tests. The good news was Willie didn't need surgery, his stomach was fine, but tests showed he was seriously diabetic.

Willie's condition was critical. He was suffering from Ketoacidosis, a life threatening condition that occurs when blood sugar isn't metabolized and the body uses stored fat for energy instead. If not treated promptly, ketones reach toxic levels in the blood and the dog dies.

That's where Willie was; his blood sugar level was through the roof, he wasn't producing insulin and he had toxic levels of ketones in his blood.

I didn't see this coming. I didn't recognize symptoms of diabetes when I saw them and now my dog was dying.

The Disease

What Is Canine Diabetes?

I knew what diabetes was in people… more or less. I had heard the term often enough, had diabetic family members and knew it had something to do with blood sugar. I even knew dogs could get diabetes, but not much more.

Diabetes Mellitus is a common disease in dogs. Golden Retrievers, German Shepherds, Miniature Schnauzers, Keeshond, and Poodles have the highest incidence of diabetes, but all breeds can be affected. Female dogs with diabetes outnumber male dogs three to one. Most diabetic dogs develop diabetes between the ages of 6 to 9 years old.

Dogs become diabetic when the islet cells in the pancreas either stop producing insulin or don't produce enough insulin. In some cases, pancreatitis can also destroy islet cells preventing insulin from being produced.

Insulin, a hormone, enables glucose to pass into the body's cells where it is used to produce energy for metabolism. Not having enough insulin results in hyperglycemia (high blood sugar) and glycosuria (high urine sugar).

The signs of diabetes include:

- Being very thirsty, drinking lots of water

- Urinating often

- Being hungry all the time

- Loosing weight

Dogs with untreated or undiagnosed diabetes are constantly thirsty and urinate often because glucose builds to high levels in their bloodstream and their kidneys work overtime flushing the excess blood sugar out of their body through their urine. Urinating large amounts of fluid causes the dog to dehydrate and increases the urge to drink large amounts of water. Dogs with untreated diabetes are often hungry and tired because their body is unable to properly produce the energy it needs.

Looking back, it's easy to recognize these symptoms now. Willie would drink half the water in his bowl at a time, go outside and urinate for fifteen minutes then come back in and do it all over again.

Our deck has four steps down to the yard. Willie always bound up these steps without missing a beat. Shortly before he was diagnosed, he would slowly climb the first two steps and rest a few moments before climbing the rest of the way up.

These are symptoms of diabetes.

Diabetes can't be cured or fixed. It can only be managed. One aspect of managing canine diabetes that can be frustrating is determining the proper insulin dose for your dog. It was pretty frustrating for Willie and me. You will work closely with your veterinarian to determine how much insulin to give your dog and how often to give it.

People with diabetes keep their blood sugar level within a very tight range. They do this by testing their blood sugar with a meter each day and use insulin to adjust their blood sugar level as needed to keep it within the proper range.

Dogs, on the other hand, aren't regulated nearly as closely as people are.

The normal blood sugar (glucose) range for dogs is 68 - 126 mg/dL. Once your veterinarian determines the initial insulin dose for your dog, you'll give your dog the prescribed dose for several days then your veterinarian will test your dogs blood sugar level again. Depending on what your dogs new blood sugar level is, your veterinarian will adjust the insulin dose if needed to bring your dogs blood sugar closer to normal levels.

If your dog responds well to insulin therapy it won't take long to determine the proper insulin dose needed to maintain your dog's blood sugar levels. Once that's done your veterinarian will test and monitor your dog's blood sugar every couple months.

On the other hand, if your dog does not respond well to insulin therapy it can take many dosage adjustments and blood sugar tests to determine the correct amount of insulin needed to properly maintain your dog's blood sugar levels.

This can be really frustrating.

Willie didn't respond well to his initial insulin therapy and had his insulin dose adjusted repeatedly. What makes it frustrating is each time Willie's dose was adjusted we would go back a few days later to test his blood sugar. The veterinarian would ask how Willie was doing and I would say Willie seemed to be doing better. His appetite seemed better, he appeared to have more energy, he was more active, it was all good. And then, more often than not, Willie's test would come back showing his blood sugar levels still way above normal.

As frustrating as it may be, stay patient, keep working with your vet because in the end, when it's finally right and everything is under control it will be worth all the effort.

Complications

The 'Mean' Disease

Diabetes has been called a 'mean' disease. It can be difficult to treat, and if not managed properly can cause many severe and critical health problems. What makes diabetes 'mean' is a long list of complications many dogs develop as they struggle with the disease.

Complications include:

- Ketoacidosis (DKA)
- Cataracts
- Uveitis and Glaucoma
- Diabetic Neuropathy
- Infection

Ketoacidosis (DKA)

Ketoacidosis is a life-threatening condition which results when the body uses fat instead of glucose (sugar) for energy.

The body uses fat for energy when there isn't enough insulin available for muscles to metabolize glucose. When muscles can't get enough glucose to use to produce the energy they need they begin to starve. When glucose isn't available for energy and muscles begin to starve they use stored fat for energy. When fat is metabolized it produces a by-product called Ketones (an acid), which is normally excreted in the urine. If the kidneys are unable to flush the excess ketones out of the body fast enough, the excess ketones will eventually reach a toxic level that causes ketoacidosis.

While the body is metabolizing fat and producing ketones, it is not using glucose. The kidneys use urine to flush the excess ketones and glucose out of the body. But as ketone and unused glucose levels rise the kidneys must produce more and more urine to use to clear the body of toxins which results in the body becoming dehydrated. It a vicious spiral that must be recognized and treated immediately.

What are the signs of ketoacidosis?

- Polyuria (excessive urination)

- Polydipsia (excessive water consumption)

- High blood-sugar levels

- High levels of ketones in the urine

- Constantly tired

- Nausea, vomiting (vomiting can be caused by many illnesses, not just ketoacidosis!)

- Abdominal pain

- Difficulty breathing (short, deep breaths)

- Acetone odor (smells like nail polish remover) or a fruity sticky sweet smell on breath

- A hard time paying attention, or confusion.

- Dehydration, (sunken eyeball, reduced tissue turgor, dry tongue)

Question: *What do you do if you think your dog is developing ketoacidosis?*

Answer: <u>*Take your dog to your veterinarian immediately!*</u>

How do you prevent ketoacidosis?

Carefully monitoring your dog is the best way of preventing ketoacidosis. There is no specific method for preventing ketoacidosis, however knowing how your dog normally behaves and functions is important. Recognizing when your dog is not behaving normally is the first step in catching ketoacidosis early.

Testing your dogs urine for sugar at home when you suspect ketoacidosis may be developing will allow you to catch it at the earliest stages before it becomes critical.

Feed your dog a low fat, low carbohydrate diet.

Be especially watchful if your dog is being treated with steroids.

Cataracts

Sadly, many diabetic dogs develop cataracts and go blind within a year of being diagnosed with diabetes. High blood sugar levels cause the eye's lens to become cloudy and opaque, leading to loss of vision in the eye.

The good news is dogs adapt very quickly to their blindness and use other senses, particularly smell and sound, much more effectively than you or I could to develop a mental map of their surroundings. Just as people who go blind soon adapt, so do dogs.

Dog owners often struggle with the idea of their dog losing its vision. Of course extra care should be taken to avoid moving furniture or leaving obstacles in their paths. But you will be amazed at how well a dog that is practically blind with cataracts can navigate it's way around the house and do so at a frightening pace too!

A blind dog can hear a can of food being opened at the other end of the house and will know what kind of food it is long before it arrives at your feet.

I was hoping we would get lucky and cataracts wouldn't be an issue for Willie. Unfortunately he developed a full cataract in his left eye and can no longer see out of that eye. Now another cataract is developing in his right eye too.

Uveitis and Glaucoma

Occasionally when a cataract develops it leaks protein into the eyeball. This causes a severe inflammation inside the eye called uveitis. If this happens your dog will need to be examined by a canine opthamologist. If left untreated, uveitis can develop into glaucoma or cause a detached retina. Vision loss is usually permanent if these conditions develop.

Diabetic Neuropathy (Peripheral Neuropathy)

High levels of blood glucose can cause nerve damage. This problem is seen more often in diabetic cats but does occur in dogs as well. Owners sometimes mistake peripheral neuropathy as a sign of old age, but it may actually be the first symptom of a diabetic dog.

The peripheral nerves make up the part of the nervous system which is outside the brain and spinal cord (the central nervous system). Neuropathy is a general term meaning dysfunction of some part of the peripheral nervous system. Typical signs of peripheral neuropathies include weakness or paralysis, reduced or absent muscle reflexes, reduced or absent muscle tone, and a loss of muscle mass. There may also be loss of pain sensation.

The first sign of peripheral neuropathy most owners notice is a weakness in their dog's hind end. The dog may stop to rest after short periods of exercise and have trouble climbing stairs. This weakness gradually affects the front legs as well. There may be coughing because the muscles around the larynx are weakened.

Megaesophagus can become a problem in some breeds. This is a chronic dilation (expansion) of the esophagus which occurs because of loss of normal muscle tone and function preventing the dog from swallowing normally. Dogs that develop megaesophagus regurgitate undigested food after meals and may develop aspiration pneumonia due to inhalation of food particles or other foreign matter.

The good news is these problems can most often be reversed when blood sugar levels are brought under control.

Infection

It is common for diabetic dogs to have recurring infections. High blood sugar levels create an ideal environment for bacterial growth. As bacteria grow and multiply they produce more glucose from cellular division causing blood glucose levels to rise even higher. It becomes a vicious cycle. Dogs with diabetes must be watched closely for signs of infection. The most common types of infection include; skin conditions, prostrate infections, urinary tract infections, and pneumonia.

Things You Need To Know About Insulin

Insulin has to be given by injection. It is a protein. If it is taken by mouth it will be digested in the stomach just like food and will be ineffective. It must be injected into the fat just under the skin, where it can be absorbed into the bloodstream.

The Right Time To Give Your Dog Insulin

Occasionally the topic of 'when is the right time to give your dog insulin' comes up. One question that gets asked more often than expected is, *"What do you do when you give your dog insulin and then it won't eat?"*

My answer to this is, unless you've been directed to do so by your vet, _never give your dog insulin before it eats_.

Always wait until after your dog has eaten before giving it insulin. Remember the reason you're giving your dog insulin is to control its blood sugar levels. When your dog eats a meal, its blood sugar levels increase. To regulate those levels you give your dog the extra insulin it needs, but isn't producing itself, to maintain its blood sugar at proper levels.

So, if you give your dog insulin before it eats, and then it doesn't eat, there won't be any excess blood sugar for the insulin you just gave your dog to regulate. The insulin is going to reduce whatever blood sugar is available and the risk of your dog becoming hypoglycemic is very high. Hypoglycemia happens when your dog's blood sugar levels drop dangerously low causing your dog to become extremely lethargic and possibly lapsing into a diabetic coma.

If this happens it's a medical emergency. Rub corn syrup on your dog's gums and get it to your veterinarian as quickly as possible for the urgent care it needs!

Remember, give your dog insulin only after it has eaten its food - not before.

Buying Insulin at Walmart

When insulin was initially prescribed for Willie, I bought it directly from the university vet school pharmacy. At the time I paid $86 for each vial of Humulin N insulin I used. At first Willie was going through two or three vials of insulin a month which got pretty expensive. Then one day I was at the vet school pharmacy getting more insulin and the pharmacist told me I could save a lot of money if I bought insulin at Walmart. He said I didn't even need a prescription. That I could walk in and buy it over-the-counter.

I left the vet school pharmacy without buying any insulin and drove to the nearest Walmart. Went to the pharmacy and told the person at the counter I needed a vial of insulin for my dog. I thought I had made a mistake because the counter clerk asked me if I had a prescription. I told her no, she said no problem and got me a vial of Humulin N insulin, the exact same stuff I was getting at the vet school pharmacy.

Price: $23.60 - a savings of over $60 on each vial of insulin!

Since I began buying Willie's insulin at Walmart the price has crept up somewhat. The last price I paid for insulin at Walmart was $26. Still a bargain!

If you're paying more than $30 a vial for your dog's insulin I suggest you check out the nearest Walmart. You maybe as pleasantly surprised as I was.

A Scary Story And A Lesson Learned

Buying insulin for Willie had become routine. I had driven to the store, stood at the pharmacy counter, asked for insulin, swiped my card and driven home so many times the process had become completely automatic by now. Buying insulin no longer required any thought. I was on auto-pilot and when the insulin vial got low, getting more insulin just happened.

One day I drove to Walmart, went to the pharmacy counter and asked for another vial of insulin for my dog. The clerk got the insulin, ringed me up and I went home. That evening Willie ate his food and I got the new vial of insulin out to give him his injection. Normally, Humulin N insulin has a milky, cloudy appearance. When I opened the new insulin I had gotten earlier that day, I immediately noticed it was crystal clear and not cloudy at all.

I should have set the vial down right then and called my veterinarian and asked about the change in appearance. I didn't. Instead after noticing the big difference in appearance I thought it must be a new, improved version of the insulin I had been giving Willie. It wasn't…

That evening I loaded the syringe with the new insulin and gave Willie his injection just like I had hundreds of times before. The next morning Willie seemed fine. I gave him his breakfast and another insulin injection. Later in the day it seemed like Willie was drinking a lot of water and needing to go out more often. And even though it seemed like he was laying around more than usual, his behavior still wasn't raising any red flags in my mind.

The next morning I came down to find Willie's water bowl empty and pools of urine all over the room. Willie was listless and lying motionless on his bed. I checked his blood sugar level and it was off the chart! Willie was in trouble!

I called my vet and told him what Willie's blood sugar reading was. He asked me if there had been any recent changes to Willie's routine. I told him nothing had changed except the new vial of insulin looked different. He asked me to read the insulin label to him. As soon as I looked at the label I knew what the problem was.

The insulin I had been giving Willie was Humulin R, not Humulin N. The pharmacy clerk had given me the wrong type of insulin and I never took the time to look at the label, even after I noticed the difference in appearance.

Humulin R is a short acting insulin and is crystal clear in appearance. It takes affect 30-60 minutes after being injected, peaks in 2-4 hours and lasts for 5-8 hours.

Humulin N, on the other hand, is an intermediate acting insulin and has a cloudy milky-white appearance. It takes affect 1-3 hours after being injected, peaks around 8 hours and lasts 12-16 hours.

My vet told me to go back to the pharmacy and get the correct insulin. When I returned, I was able to get Willie to eat some food for his breakfast and gave him the correct insulin. I watched him closely, monitored his blood sugar and sent my vet email updates throughout the day. By the end of the following day he was back to normal.

This crisis could have easily been avoided if I hadn't been so careless. It's easy to settle into a routine, become complacent and not pay attention to details.

The lesson learned is to always check and read the label of any medication you're giving to your dog, your child, yourself or to anyone. If something looks wrong - STOP. Question it, investigate, call someone, check and re-check until you're satisfied you are making the right decision. It's much better to take a little time to be sure everything is correct and proper than to regret a decision made in haste later.

Other Important Things To Know About Insulin...

Insulin won't work if it is stored below 36 degrees or above 86 degrees.

Don't leave vials of insulin in a car on hot or cold days.

Insulin can also be damaged by sunlight. Keep it out of direct sunlight.

If you plan on flying to a destination, keep your dogs insulin in your carry-on luggage. Do not put your dogs insulin in your checked luggage where it will be placed in the cargo hold and may get too hot or cold.

It is important to make sure the insulin is well mixed. But you do not want to shake the vial or over agitate the insulin when mixing. Over agitating insulin can cause any of the following problems:

- Insulin threads/clumps can form reducing the overall effective amount of insulin in the vial, thus reducing the number of doses available from that vial.

- Frosting - over agitation of insulin - can cause insulin to stick to the vial, "frosting" it like ice on a window. This frosting may not even be visible to the naked eye but it reduces the effective amount of insulin in the vial.

- Micro bubbles can form in the vial and when drawn into the syringe reduce the amount of insulin in the dose.

Micro bubbles aren't a major problem unless you shake the vial so much that the liquid is "foaming" and you immediate draw a dose from the vial. Clumps and frosting are much more serious issues that can seriously affect the effectiveness of an insulin dose.

The safest method of mixing insulin is to gently roll the vial back and forth between the palms of your hands, tilting your hands from side-to-side to move the fluid around the entire vial. Be sure you gently roll the vial enough times to ensure the insulin is thoroughly mixed.

Giving Injections

Diabetic dogs need insulin, and they get it by you injecting insulin under their skin with a syringe. Your veterinarian will show you how to give the injection when insulin is initially prescribed. Giving an injection isn't hard to do and most people develop good injection skills quickly.

Massaging or stroking your dog before an injection calms them and helps them from being surprised by the needle stick. An extra minute or two of petting and relaxing may be all your dog needs to prepare for an injection.

Many people reward their dog with food during or just after injection time. Giving the injection while the dog is busy eating is very common. Putting a small treat in front of your dog can help keep them still for an injection. Some people give a treat right after the injection. The dog is well behaved during the injection because it knows a treat is coming. A big hug and praise after an injection is always comforting and maybe all your dog needs.

Always warm the insulin before injecting it into your dog. Human diabetics say injecting cold insulin is uncomfortable, this is no doubt true for dogs too. Insulin at room temperature is far more comfortable than cold insulin when injected. After filling the syringe with the proper amount of insulin, hold the syringe between your fingers for a minute. Some people take the entire vial of insulin out of the refrigerator and let it sit until it is room temperature. It is probably better to warm only the amount needed for each injection and place the insulin vial back into the refrigerator as soon as possible.

** IMPORTANT! **
DO NOT USE HOT WATER, A MICROWAVE OR ANYTHING OTHER THAN YOUR HANDS TO WARM INSULIN!

Before giving Willie his injection, I warm my hands with a cup of hot coffee or tea then hold his syringe between the palms of my hands for a few minutes to warm the insulin up.

Use the heat from your hands to warm the insulin or let the syringe (or vial) sit out at room temperature for a few minutes.

When you are ready to inject the insulin, push the needle quickly and firmly through the skin. Going through the skin is the most sensitive time. Once the needle is through the skin your dog doesn't feel much.

Once the needle is in, inject the insulin at a moderate rate. Not too fast and not too slow. After a few injections you'll know what you're doing, in the mean time your dog will let you know if you are doing it right.

No need to use alcohol wipes. Most people do not clean the injection site with alcohol before an injection. Alcohol doesn't "disinfect" the skin, it only wets the fur and may cause stinging during the injection. Unless your dog is very dirty you don't need to clean the injection site.

Disposable insulin syringes are meant to be used one time only. Most syringes needles have a coating that helps the needle go in easier and more comfortably. Each time the needle is used a portion of the coating is worn away causing the needle to slide less smoothly if it is used again.

Please use a new insulin syringe
each time you give your dog an injection.

The needles are extremely thin and the point on the tip of the needle is easily twisted or bent. In fact, every time the needle is used the tip of the needle becomes twisted or bent to some degree. Reusing a needle can cause skin damage and cause the injection site to heal more slowly. Please always use a new syringe each time you inject your dog.

The following three photos illustrate how delicate the point of an insulin needle is:

Brand new, unused insulin needle.

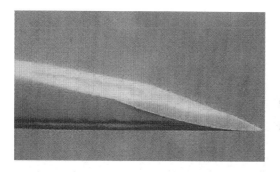

Insulin needle used once.

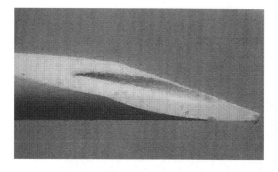

Insulin needle used twice.

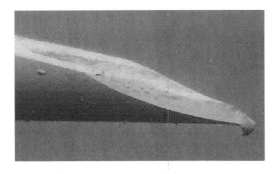

If your dog is extremely sensitive to injections you might try using an anesthetic like Orajel or Ambesol to help make injections more comfortable. Rub a little Orajel on your dog's skin where you will be injecting the insulin. Wait a couple minutes for the Orajel to numb the skin then inject the insulin as usual.

Some people are afraid of needles. If you are one of them you need to learn to be comfortable and confident using a syringe. Start by taking an empty syringe and hold it in your hand. Become familiar with how it feels. Pull the plunger out and push it back in over and over again. Get use to how that motion feels. Practice giving an injection to a piece of fruit or a stuffed animal. The more you practice the more confident you will become. Your goal is to push the needle into your dog's skin quickly but gently and inject the insulin in one smooth motion. It may feel clumsy at first, but keep practicing and you will quickly gain confidence in your technique.

Remember, if you are concerned about hurting your dog while giving an injection your dog may sense your fear and become nervous. Relax. Step back and take a deep breath or two. Insulin syringes use very small, thin needles that don't hurt much, if at all.

It is important to use a different spot on your dog's body each time you give an injection. Ask your veterinarian to show the best places on your dog to give injections. Every dog is different. A good spot for one dog can be a very sensitive area for another. Most owners are advised to give their dogs injections in the same general area of the body such as on the side behind the shoulder or the hind end. Different parts of the body absorb insulin faster than others. Just avoid injecting in the exact same spot each time. Injecting in different parts of the body will prevent one spot from becoming too sore.

After an injection you might notice a tiny bit of the insulin leaking out of the injection site. It shouldn't happen very often but is normal and shouldn't be a problem. Consult your veterinarian if you are concerned your dog is not getting a full dose of insulin.

It is possible to make a mistake giving an injection. If you notice any of the following things it may mean some or all of the insulin may not have gotten injected properly:

• Your dog's fur is wet with insulin

- You can smell the distinct odor of the insulin. Humulin NPH has a unique odor and can easily be detected on your dog's fur.

- Your fingers are wet with insulin.

If you think you blew an injection, call your veterinarian to discuss what you should do next. It is not safe to try and guess how much insulin was injected. In this situation it's usually best not to give a replacement shot. Wait until it is time to give the next shot and give the usual dose of insulin. Missing one scheduled injection is not the end of the world. Your dog's blood sugar may be high for a few hours but that's a lot safer than giving it too much insulin.

Discuss with your veterinarian ahead of time what you should do if you make a mistake while injecting your dog so you will be prepared if it ever happens.

Injection Quick Tips

- Do not use an alcohol swab before the injection.

- Use a different spot each time you inject your dog.

- Relax. Spend a little time petting or massaging your dog before giving the injection.

- Pinch and pull your dog's skin up occasionally

throughout the day so he won't always see it as a warning he's about to get stuck.

- Use positive reinforcement. Give the injection while your dog is eating or give him a treat after the injection.

- Always warm the insulin up before giving the injection.

- Hold the syringe parallel to your dog's body while pushing the needle in.

- Be calm and your dog will be calm as well.

Hypoglycemia

Hypoglycemia is a sudden drop in your dog's blood glucose level. When your dog goes "hypo" it has a critically low level of blood glucose which can cause serious brain damage or death. *It can occur in diabetic dogs when too much insulin has been given.*

Hypoglycemic symptoms include:

- Depression/Lethargy

- Confusion/Dizziness

- Trembling

- Ataxia (loss of coordination and/or balance)

- Loss of excretory or bladder control

- Vomiting then loss of consciousness and/or seizures

- Sleepiness/Unresponsiveness (An important, easy to miss sign that your dog's blood glucose levels are getting too low is when you call your dog and it fails to respond or is slow to respond.)

- Dog becoming more vocal can be a symptom of hypoglycemia.

As soon as you determine your dog is having a hypoglycemic episode, rub corn syrup on it's gums (even if the dog is unconscious, but not while its having a seizure) and take it immediately to your veterinarian. Take the corn syrup with you and continue rubbing it on your dog's gums until you get to your veterinarian's office.

The best place to apply corn syrup is sublingually, rub corn syrup under your dog's tongue. There is a high concentration of blood vessels under the tongue that enables rapid absorption of the corn syrup into your dog's system.

NEVER try to make a seizing or unconscious dog swallow!

Trying to give a seizing or unconscious dog food or liquid can cause it to choke. It is also possible for the dog to aspirate (inhale into the lungs instead of swallowing) whatever you are trying to give it causing other serious problems.

Monitoring Your Dog

Until your dog's diabetes is regulated, and even after, it's important to monitor its blood sugar levels closely. Monitoring blood sugar levels can be done a couple of ways:

1) Using test strips and a glucose meter
2) Using urine glucose test strips

Glucose Meters

Probably the most common and accurate method of monitoring blood sugar levels is by using a glucose meter. This is commonly done by testing a small drop of the dog's blood with a special test strip and glucose meter several times a day. To do this correctly, you'll need a glucose meter made for dogs.

So why do you need a dog specific glucose meter? Because your blood and your dog's blood is not exactly the same. There are differences in the ratios of glucose in plasma and red blood cells between human blood and dog blood. Humans only have 58% of glucose in plasma. Your dog on the other hand, has 87.5% of glucose in plasma. This is significantly higher. If you use a glucose meter made for humans to read your dog's blood sugar, the human meter (which has been calibrated to calculate glucose levels using human glucose distributions) will give inaccurate readings which could result in you giving your dog the wrong amount of insulin.

Always use a glucose meter specifically calibrated for dogs to ensure accurate readings.

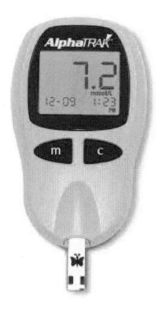

If you decide to use a glucose meter to monitor your dog you'll need to know how to draw a drop of blood from your dog. Blood for monitoring is typically drawn by pricking your dog's lip with a lancet then touching the test strip to the droplet and reading the results from the meter. Your vet will show you how to lance your dog's lip to get blood for the meter.

When I began monitoring Willie's blood sugar, I started out using a glucose meter. I wanted my readings to be as accurate as possible so I would check Willie's levels three or four times a day. I didn't like monitoring with the meter and I don't think Willie enjoyed it much either. I just couldn't get comfortable lancing Willie's lip each time I needed to check his blood sugar. It created a lot of stress for both of us so I stopped using the glucose meter and started using a different method to monitor Willie's blood sugar.

Urine Glucose Test Strips

Compared to glucose meters, urine testing is much easier and more convenient for most people, but it's a lot less accurate. Whenever the glucose level in your dog's blood rises above about 180 milligrams per deciliter (mg/dL) your dog will get rid of the excess glucose through its urine. You can measure the amount of glucose in your dog's urine by using inexpensive test strips. These test strips are most commonly sold under the brand names Diastix and Ketodiastix and can be purchased at most pharmacies.

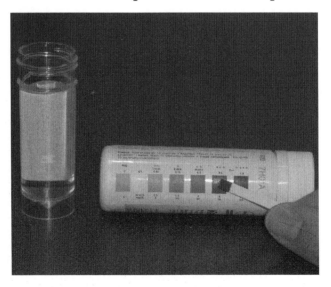

You'll need to collect a small amount of your dog's urine to test its blood sugar with a urine test strip. There are a lot of creative ways to collect dog urine. Some of the more popular methods involve Tupperware, soup ladles, saucers, mugs, etc., you name it. Or, if you're lucky enough to have a cooperative dog, you can hold the test strip directly in the stream of urine. The good news is you only need to collect a very small amount of urine for testing.

As it worked out, the best time to get a sample from Willie was when I let him out first thing in the morning. He would go outside, still half asleep, and I would follow behind him. I used a plastic 8x8 inch container that was 1 inch tall and perfect for the job. When he found a spot I would gently slide the plastic container underneath him to get a small sample. It was very easy to collect the small amount of urine needed for the test and Willie was oblivious to the entire process.

Once you have a sample of urine to test, typically you dip the test strip in the sample, wait a short period of time then match the color of the test strip to a color scale on the test strip bottle to read the glucose value. It sounds a lot more difficult than it actually is.

Urine testing is an inexpensive and easy way to do basic blood sugar monitoring and is the method I have been using to monitor Willie's blood sugar since I stopped using the glucose meter. As mentioned above, it isn't nearly as accurate or precise as monitoring with a glucose meter, but it provides an easy method of monitoring Willie's general blood sugar levels. More importantly it still allows me to catch and treat problems early before they turn into a crisis or emergency situation.

If your vet is like mine, she won't rely completely on your home monitoring to keep track of your dog's well-being. Instead she'll want to run her own glucose curve on your dog from time to time. This is a good thing, and if you haven't recently updated your dog's daily blood sugar information with your vet then this is a perfect time to review your records with her.

I want to mention something I noticed when I took Willie into the vets for a glucose curve. Whenever the vet ran a glucose curve on Willie at the vets office, his results were always higher than the results I got when I tested Willie at home. The first few times this happened I thought Willie was having an episode or was unregulated. But the more I thought about it I realized Willie would get stressed out whenever I took him in for a glucose curve. His stress level caused his blood sugar levels to elevate and result in higher than normal readings. I discussed this with my vet who said it is entirely possible for that to happen. Don't be afraid to compare your home test results with your vets results and to point out and discuss any significant differences in results.

Getting Organized

Ok, you've been testing or are just starting to test your dogs blood sugar levels, you'll want someway to record your readings.

Recording your dogs blood sugar levels can be as simple or as technologically sophisticated as you'd like it to be. There are a lot of options.

Pen and Paper

The simplest way to record your readings is with a pen and pad of paper. It's handy, inexpensive, easy to use and there's no training required.

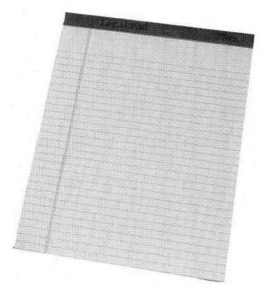

There are at least three pieces of information you will want to recored each time you test your dogs blood sugar levels:

- Date
- Time
- Blood Sugar Reading

You can track as much information as you think is necessary, but the date, time and reading are three important pieces of information you and your vet will most certainly need.

Other items that might be useful to track include:

- **Amount Of Insulin Given With Each Injection**
  Normally (until your vet tells you to do differently) this amount stays that same each time you give your dog insulin, but there could be instances where you alter the amount of insulin given. For example, when we were trying to determine the proper dose of insulin for Willie before we got him regulated there were times I would change the amount given by half a unit. I would do this when monitoring showed the previous dose was causing his levels to dip too low so I would adjust the amount given in the next injection and monitor his levels closely. Of course I did not do this without discussing it with Willie's vet first and getting her approval to do so.

- **Your Dogs Weight**

  Recording your dogs weight once a week can be useful information. Especially if your dog is obese and you're trying to help it lose weight. Recording its steady weight loss - or lack of - can be critical in developing a proper diet for your dog.

- **Water Consumption**

  Excessive water consumption is a well known symptom of diabetes. Monitoring your dogs water consumption between blood sugar tests can be a helpful indication of whether your dogs therapy is being effective. You can make a graduated water bowl or pick one up at most pet supply stores. Record the amount of water your dog drinks between blood sugar tests or at any other interval you prefer.

- **Diet Information; Amount And Type of Food**

  A diabetic dogs diet is critical to managing its disease. It is highly useful to record what your dog eats and how much food you give it at each meal. If you're giving your dog store bought food, record the amount you give, brand name, food type and tear off the nutritional information from the bag or label to keep with your notes. If you make your own dog food, record all the ingredients and recipe used along with the amount of food given at each feeding.

- **Exercise And Play**

  Believe it or not, but too much rigorous exercise can cause hypoglycemia in a diabetic dog. It may be useful to record when, for how long and what kind of exercise your dog gets. Keep notes on your dogs activity level and how engaged it is during the exercise and play time. Pay special attention to how it behaves after exercise, especially if the activity was strenuous or at a high energy level.

- **General Behavior And Activity**

  If possible, take time to observe your dog throughout the day. Do its ears perk up when you walk into the room? Does it get up and walk over to you when you sit down in your chair? Does your dog look at you when you speak to it? Will it follow you around the house or yard? Is it alert and attentive or does it seem uninterested and lethargic? Be watchful especially an hour or so after giving it an insulin injection. This is generally about the time insulin will start to take affect. Too much insulin will cause blood sugar levels to drop too low and your dog could become hypoglycemic. If that happens it might act confused, stagger around when it tries to walk or act like a rag doll and be lethargic and non-responsive. Record the date, time, reason for concern and circumstances of any behavior that concerns you.

Use A Spreadsheet

If you have a computer you might consider using a spreadsheet.

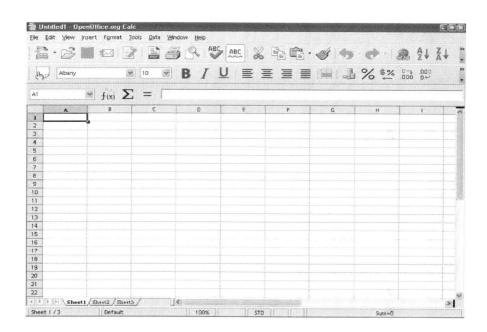

You can track everything mentioned above with a spreadsheet plus you'll be able to create very useful charts, graphs and reports you can either print out to share or email directly to your vet.

The spreadsheet you use doesn't need to be very complicated or sophisticated. Keep it simple. If you have some experience using spreadsheets then you probably already have all the skill you need to design and create something useful that will suit your needs.

On the other hand, if you don't have the time or skill to create your own spreadsheet, there's an easy solution that will get you up and running quickly. Go to your favorite search engine and search for:

"free diabetic spreadsheet template"

You'll quickly discover hundreds and thousands of organizations and people who have already created spreadsheets to log and monitor diabetic information you can use for free.

The spreadsheets you'll find searching run from the simplest, most basic to extremely complex, multi-sheet analytical systems. There are so many free diabetic spreadsheets available you'll need to spend a little time sifting through what's out there to find the perfect one that's just right for you.

Online Diabetes Logs

Another option for organizing and recording your dog's information are online diabetes logs. These are web based applications you access over the web with your browser.

Just like the free spreadsheets above, these web based apps can be very simple or quite complicated.

Here are several you can check out:

- sugarstats.com
- glucosebuddy.com
- best4diabetes.com
- glucosegraph.com
- plasmaglucose.com
- mendosa.com
- mydiabeteshome.com

Virtually all online apps provide reports and graphs you can print out to share or some apps will let you email reports directly to your vet. Even better, consider giving your vet access to your online log so they can access your dog's information whenever they need it.

And who knows, your vet may already have their own electronic medical records system with an Internet patient portal that will allow you to record your dogs information directly into a log at the vets office. Talk to your vet to see if that's an option as well.

Smartphone Apps

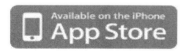 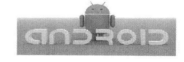

Diabetic smartphone apps make tracking your dogs blood sugar information about as easy and convenient as it can get. Since my smartphone is always with me whenever I check Willie's blood sugar levels, I can enter his numbers quickly and easily right on the spot as I take the reading. And I can even do it with one hand!

As you might imagine, there are a lot of diabetes applications available for both iPhone and Android smartphone users. Some do more, some do less and some work better than others. Below are four popular smartphone apps that are well rated:

- Glucose Buddy by Azumio
- Glucose Companion by Maxwell Software
- Diabetes Pal by Telcare, Inc.
- Diabetes Log by Distal Thoughts

Remember, *always backup your data*. A smartphone is a handheld computer that stores your data in electronic memory that can become corrupt or otherwise unusable. Always have a current backup of your data!

Exercise And Diet

Normally, unless your dog has a physical problem, exercise is good for both diabetic dogs and their owners.

Willie had always been pretty sedentary. He spends most of his days lying by my desk in my office while I work. As a result he was over weight and out of shape which most likely contributed to the diabetes he developed. Even so, exercising after the fact is still better than not exercising at all.

We began our exercise routine walking to the end of our driveway and back to the front porch. About forty feet each way. We'd get to the end of the driveway, stop and rest for a short time, then slowly walk the forty feet back to the house.

It's important to begin exercising slow and easy. You can cause hypoglycemia by exercising your dog too rigorously. Start out slow and easy. Gently increase the level of exercise as your dog gets stronger.

Be patient, don't over do it!

Willie and I have a set time each day we head out for our walk. As he got stronger and healthier we increased the distance we walked. It wasn't too long before we were walking around the block.

Diet

Your dogs diet plays an important role in managing its disease. The typical preferred diet for a diabetic dog is a low fat, low carbohydrate meal.

Some people prefer making their own dog food while others are fine using store bought food. However, **each dog is an individual and has its own unique dietary needs and requirements**. It is important to discuss your dogs diet with your vet to ensure it gets the proper food and nutrition it needs and that you are giving it the proper amount.

Many diabetic dogs are obese. Their eating schedule and food portions must be strictly controlled in order for them to loose weight. Additionally, the proper type of food must be given to maintain a balanced and healthy diet.

I considered making Willies food instead of buying it from the store. I was thinking that whatever I made had to be a lot better than anything I could possibly buy at the store. I did some research but in the end decided not to make Willies food after all. If you search the web, you'll find a number of recipes for making your own diabetic dog food that maybe just fine. I just wasn't comfortable using a generic dog food or meal recipe that wasn't specifically made for Willie.

A proper diet for a diabetic dog is not a trivial matter

and is critically important to your dogs health and well being. I decided to go with whatever food Willies vet recommended.

Willie was obese and required a special diet. His vet calculated how many calories he needed each day. We then looked at the portions and combinations of foods needed to provide a well balanced diet that would allow him to loose weight at the same time. After some trial and error, we ended up with a combination of one cup of dry dog food mixed with one quarter cup of canned dog food Willie enjoys eating. He has a meal every twelve hours and gets an insulin injection immediately following his meal.

After having Willie on the dry/canned dog food diet for six weeks, we still weren't getting the results we needed so Willies vet switched him to a prescription diet. It is more expensive but is providing the effective weigh management Willie needs right now.

Remember... before starting any exercise program, even walking forty feet to the end of the driveway, or changing your dog's diet, always talk to your veterinarian first before doing anything that may affect the health and well-being of your dog!

33 Important Questions To Ask Your Veterinarian

It is important for you to understand how your dog is being treated, how the therapy affects your dog and what to do in an emergency or when something unplanned and unexpected happens. Discussing these things ahead of time with your veterinarian will provide you with loads of peace-of-mind down the road... trust me.

Your veterinarian should be happy to take all the time necessary to discuss your dog's condition, thoroughly explain the therapy and answer all your questions. Good communication is essential. It is very important to ask your veterinarian to explain things so you understand completely. You must have a clear understanding of what's going on so you can provide the care your dog will need.

33 questions to ask your veterinarian:

1. Ask your veterinarian how much experience they have treating diabetic dogs. Having little or no experience doesn't necessarily disqualify them from treating your dog. They may be fine. However, if you are not comfortable with your veterinarian's level of experience don't hesitate to ask for a referral to a veterinarian with more experience.

2. Ask your veterinarian if they consult or work with a veterinary ophthalmologist. Diabetic dogs especially,

are prone to developing diabetic cataracts and may need to be evaluated by a specialist.

3. Does your veterinarian have an emergency number you can call? What is it?

4. Ask your veterinarian what to do if there is an emergency after hours (nights and weekends)?

5. Is there another clinic or veterinarian your veterinarian refers patients to when they are on vacation? What is the name, address and phone number of that clinic?

6. How will diabetes affect your dog's other health conditions, if any?

7. Will insulin adversely react with any other medication your dog is taking?

8. What other health problems should you be watching for? (i.e., Cataracts? Infections?)

9. Are there any kind of records you should keep to help your veterinarian evaluate your dog's condition and progress? Some dog owners keep a notebook documenting each insulin dose, time of injection, notes about eating, results of any home urine or blood glucose testing, and other observations like vomiting, diarrhea, lethargy.

10. What is the best way to monitor your dog's condition at home? (i.e., monitoring water consumption, watching for excessive thirst, urination, hunger, weight gain or loss, lethargy, urine sugar, ketones in urine, blood glucose monitoring)

11. How often will your veterinarian want to check your dog's progress until its diabetes is under control? Weekly, every other week, once a month?

12. How will your veterinarian determine how well your dog's diabetes is being controlled? Your observations, blood tests done at the veterinarian's office?

13. Will a blood glucose curve be necessary (testing the blood glucose every hour or two for a full day)?

14. When your dog's diabetes is under control, how often will your veterinarian check your dog's condition? Monthly, every 3-4 months? What tests will your veterinarian use to evaluate you dog's condition?

15. How much should you budget for testing, checkups, etc.? How much should you reasonably expect to spend on your dog's health care each month?

16. How important is it to give your dog its insulin injection at a certain time each day?

17. How long after your dog eats can you wait to give the injection before it's necessary to adjust the dose?

18. If its necessary to give the injection later than the answer to question 17 above, what do you do?

- Do you skip this shot or do you give less insulin (how much less)?
- Do you give the next shot at the regular time?

19. What do you do if you think you missed giving a shot or gave an incomplete shot but you're not sure? Do you give another shot?

20. What should you do if your dog vomits after you've given the insulin injection?

21. How much insulin should you give your dog if it won't eat its meal?

22. How much insulin should you give your dog if it only eats part of its meal?

23. You fed your dog but forgot to give the insulin shot. What do you do?

24. What if your dog eats extra food, candy, or garbage. Should you give your dog extra insulin?

25. Your dog didn't act like it was feeling well last night and doesn't look 'right' this morning either. Do you give your dog its regular dose of insulin?

This has been discussed earlier, but is important enough to mention again.

Hypoglycemia is an emergency for your dog!

Be sure you understand what it is, how to recognize when your dog goes 'hypo' and how you should respond. Ask your veterinarian to explain hypoglycemia (low blood sugar) and how serious it is.

Always have corn syrup (Karo) or another source of sugar available (pancake syrup, honey) to use if needed. Also know that many dogs will not show any signs of hypoglycemia, even when their blood glucose is very low.

26. What are the physical signs of hypoglycemia? How will your dog act when it is hypoglycemic?

27. What does your veterinarian want you to do if you think your dog is hypoglycemic?

28. Your dog looks sleepy and is lethargic. What should you do? Do you give food or Karo? How much?

29. Your dog is wobbling around, stumbling and whining strangely. What do you do?

30. Your dog is having a seizure or is unconscious. What do you do?

31. If you think your dog is hypoglycemic, when is it reasonable to call the veterinarian and under what conditions should you immediately take your dog to the veterinarian or emergency clinic?

32. What should you do if your dog's breath has a strange chemical smell?

33. Can your dog continue its normal physical activities like going on walks, running, swimming, etc.?

Lifestyle Changes

Diabetes changed my relationship with Willie.

It made it better.

Before Willie was diagnosed with diabetes we played and went on walks but I didn't pay as much attention to him then as I do now. This has been the biggest lifestyle change since Willie became a diabetic.

Now, I know how he behaves when he's feeling good and how he behaves when he's feeling bad. I'm 'tuned in' and recognize his subtle, non-verbal signals I wasn't aware of before. I know when he comes up to me if he wants to play or just a rub behind the ear. Developing a wonderful relationship with Willie, unlike any I've had with any other dog, has been the biggest joy I've received from this experience. He is my constant companion and friend.

Another lifestyle change has been adapting to his schedule. Willie eats every twelve hours and must have an insulin injection immediately after his meal. There's not a lot of room to deviate from the schedule. We stick to it and avoid problems.

Occasionally I travel for work. When its necessary for me to go out of town I spend extra time with the techs where I board Willie to be sure they understand the level of care

Willie needs and how to give it to him. I make sure they have my contact info as well as the contact info for the veterinarian who treated Willie at the university veterinary hospital.

The other lifestyle change we both benefit greatly from is our regular exercise and play schedule. We take time almost every day to walk, play and horse around for at least an hour. Both of us have lost weight and eat better. Sadly, I'm not sure I would have started walking or exercising if not for Willie's diabetes.

Acquiring a disease is never good. It can make you pause, reassess and discover opportunities for a richer, more fulfilling life. If you are living with a diabetic dog, take advantage of these moments. I assure you, the love and companionship you will enjoy is beyond measure.

Last Word

Thank you for reading my book!

I hope you found this information helpful and encouraging. Canine diabetes doesn't have to be the debilitating, life ending disease it so often turns out to be for many dogs. Understanding canine diabetes and your loving care will ensure you and your dog enjoy each others companionship for a long time to come!

If you enjoyed this book please tell your friends about it.

I am always grateful when my readers leave thoughtful and sincere reviews of my books. If you enjoyed this book please consider leaving a short review on the site you got the book from. I appreciate your encouragement and kind words more than you will know, and your comments help other readers as well.

Best wishes to you and your dog -
Amy Newton Thomas

Postscript

It's been more than two years since Willie was taken to the emergency room at the university vet school. When I saw him that day, so close to dying, I would never have dreamed he would be sitting here beside me today.

We've had to make some changes and learn some new routines. But in the larger scheme of things the inconveniences have been minor compared to the gift of more time with a good dog.

I hope and wish the best for you and your dog too.
Amy Newton Thomas

We invite you to connect:
twitter/amynewtonthomas
twitter/brucepea
www.brucepea.com/lwdd

Homemade Dog Food
Clean + delicious